I0442019

Anti-Inflammatory Essential Oils
By Eve Bell

Copyright © 2015 Eve Bell
All Rights Reserved
The information provided in this book is for educational and entertainment
purposes only. The reader is responsible for his or her own actions and the author
does not accept any responsibilities for any liabilities or damages, real or perceived,
resulting from the use of this information.

You'll learn in this book:

Get control of your inflammation

Whether it's due to arthritis, an old sports injury or another cause entirely, there are ways to manage and reverse inflammation using Aromatherapy. Essential oils are flexible in the way you can prepare and implement them, and they only take seconds to apply. In this Ebook, you will learn:

- What causes inflammation?
- What essential oils are?
- The different preparations you will be making.
- How to mix and apply them.
- Uses for essential oils to treat acute swelling as well as chronic swelling.
- Which preparations are most beneficial for treating inflammation?
- How often they should be used.

Introduction

If you are reading this eBook, you are on your way to learning one holistic method of reducing your inflammation. Essential oils have been used for centuries for a myriad of conditions, and will benefit you as well. I will walk you through the basics, explain how they work, and also show you how to mix your own remedies.

Chapter 1: The story on inflammation

One of the easiest ways to begin treating a condition is to know what causes it. Getting to the root of the matter, the basis of holistic healing, will allow your body to heal itself efficiently and the way nature intended.

What is it?

It is the body's immediate response to injury. Like an airbag in a vehicle, tissues swell to protect the injured body part from incurring more damage. This starts the healing process. It also protects the inner tissues from infection by pushing any infectious materials out of the body.

For instance, if you get a splinter that you cannot extract and it gets infected, the inflammation does not allow the splinter go to deeper into the skin. It, in reality, pushes the white blood cells (puss) along with the splinter to the surface of the skin so you can take it out. When you do not address the issue that is causing the inflammation, it has a chance to worsen, leading to other diseases. There are different stages of inflammation:

Acute Inflammation

This type of inflammation usually occurs rapidly upon most injuries and persists for a few days. If you have ever had difficulty swallowing after coughing while you have a cold, it is because of inflammation. Puffiness around a cut on the skin or ingrown toenail is also acute inflammation. If dermatitis is left untreated, it can become inflamed.

More severe cases of acute inflammation are the inflamed membranes of the lungs which causes bronchitis. There is also inflammation of the sinus cavities. Very intense exercise or overdoing it during an exercise regimen that your body is not used to doing can also cause acute inflammation.

Chronic Inflammation

This is inflammation that persists for months and in many cases, years. It can lead to debilitating diseases such as rheumatoid arthritis, emphysema, and endometriosis.
Chronic swelling is also present in severe cases of sinusitis and Crohn's disease. It also contributes to Irritable Bowel Syndrome and peptic ulcers as well. Tuberculosis is also directly linked to chronic swelling of the alveoli in the lungs.

Not all swelling is bad.

Swelling that is related to minor cuts and bruising is not bad. It just means your body is padding the injury so it heals without further trauma. It will go down on its own. Swelling with redness, soreness, and is filling or is filled with puss is infected. This means that the infection must be dealt with before it worsens and leads to other complications.

Chapter 2: What are essential oils?

Essential oils are the true essence of the plant. It is the unadulterated oil that you can get from either the leaves, or flowers of the plants or the rind of fruit. They are often mixed with carrier oils like Sweet Almond, Apricot Kernel, and Grapeseed to produce massage oils, mineral salts for baths, and even toxin-free cleaners for the home.

They are integral part of aromatherapy, meaning they are the main constituent. Essential oils have been used to treat everything from colds and flu to arthritis and other inflammatory diseases. Many of the oils are completely safe and can be used while taking already existing medications.

Essential oils in a diffuse can calm nerves and quiet anxiety attacks. Essential oils in other blends can be used to reduce fevers swelling and even treat skin conditions.

Before you start using essential oils, you have to make sure that you are not sensitive to them. They are very concentrated forms of the herbs, and they can cause rashes and other skin irritations.

The best way to prevent this is to perform a patch test. Your local herb shop will have samples of essential oils and they can assist you in a patch test. During a patch test, one drop of essential oil is added to ¼ teaspoon of base carrier oil and then placed on a small patch of skin.

If you are sensitive, the irritation can appear anywhere from immediately, if you are very sensitive skin, up to 24 hours later. It is always best to wait the 24 hours just to be sure.

Essential oils evaporate in high heat. Keep any blends and preparations in a cool dark place with tight lids. Once they are made into preparations, they have a 3 month self-life before their effectiveness begins to diminish.

You can use essential oils in many preparations:

Massage oil

- Add 6 drops of essential oils to one tablespoon of carrier oil or carrier oil blend.
- If you are making 4 ounces of a carrier oil mixture, add 50 drops of essential oils.

Bath Salts and Mineral Baths

- These are essential oils that have been mixed with carrier oils and then added to a blend of borax, baking soda and sea salts. If you suffer from hypertension or other heart conditions, you can substitute ground oatmeal for the salt to make your mineral bath.

Lotions

- You can add essential oils to plain, lotion to make lotion-based massage oil or lotion for the skin.

Shampoos and Liquid body soaps

- Essential oils can be added to existing shampoos and body soaps to treat inflamed skin due to dermatitis, eczema and other skin conditions.

Poultices/Masks

- These are made when essential oils are added to herbal pastes or facial clary or mud.

- These are often implemented for immediate treatment.

There are other preparations, but the ones listed above are the most effective for anti-inflammatory purposes.

It is best to use glass, porcelain, and wooden tools to make the preparations so as not to change the chemical make-up of the essential oils. Never heat essential oils in order to make a preparation.

If you want to add them to salves or other preparations that require heating, wait until the preparation is almost cool, but you are still able to stir in the essential oils. This will make sure that the essential oils will not evaporate.

Chapter 3: Your anti-inflammatory essential oils

Though there are many essential oils on the market, when you go looking for those that specifically treat swelling, and tighten muscles and other causes of inflammation, you narrow the playing field considerably.

To be able to treat any ailment that causes inflammation effectively, you're going to need the following essential oils.

DON'T USE IF YOU'RE PREGNANT!

Lavender (avendulan angustifolia)

- This is essential oil is a very versatile and affordable essential oil that should be a staple in every home.
- It reduces inflammation, fights infection, and speeds the healing of wounds. It also lessens the pain of lumbago, rheumatism, muscular aches and sprains.

Peppermint (mentha piperita)

- When treating swelling caused by a bact
  infection, using peppermint essential oil
  attack the bacteria causing the infection.
- It also has anaesthetic blends that treat swell
  with intense pain, like rheumatoid arthritis.
- Not to be used during the latter part of pregnan
  It has been known to diminish breast milk.

Roman Chamomile (Chamaemelum nobile)

- This essential oil has been used for centuries to bring down swelling, sooth inflamed joints, and to treat arthritis, even rheumatoid arthritis.

Cinnamon leaf (cinnamomum zeylanicum)

- This essential oil is mainly used to bring down swelling and increase circulation, speeding healing. It does have warming properties to help loosen tight muscles.
- Don't use this oil in a blend before bedtime. It is a stimulant and will cause you to have difficulty falling asleep.

DO NOT USE THE BARK ESSENTIAL OIL. IT IS HIGHLY TOXIC. THIS OIL IS ONLY TO BE USED IN MORE SEVERE INFLAMMATION CASES.

Black Pepper (piper nigrum)

- This essential oil is used in most blends to treat arthritis, muscular aches and pains, rheumatic pain, sprains and stiffness.
- This oil is also a stimulant and should not be used before bedtime.
- The heat produced by black pepper can loosen tight muscles and relieve intense pain.

French Basil (ocimum basilicum)

- Included in first aid blends, it reduces swelling, and soothes the aches and pains due to injuries and inflammation.
- It has also been used to treat rheumatism.

Yarrow (achillea millefolium)

- This essential oil is incorporated in blends that reduce inflammation and help to treat arteriosclerosis, thrombosis, and rheumatoid arthritis.

Camphor (cinnamomum camphora)

- The white camphor is the only one that is used in aromatherapy as the brown and yellow are toxic.
- It is added to blends that reduce inflammation and target sprains and rheumatoid arthritis.
- This is another stimulant.

Tumeric (curcuma longa)

- The powered form of the herb has a notoriety all its own, but the essential oil is used in blends to target rheumatoid arthritis. It also helps to reduce muscle aches and helps to alleviate pain.

Sweet Marjoram (origanum marjorana)

- This essential oil is used to treat mainly injuries that cause swelling such as arthritis, lumbago, muscular aches and stiffness, rheumatism as well as sprains and muscle strain.

The mildest carrier oils are Sweet Almond oil and Apricot Kernel oil. To help reduce inflammation, you can add grape seed oil to the blend as well.

Chapter 4: Sprains

The ligaments that connect your bones to one another can become torn, causing a sprain. The worse the tear, the more intense the pain and the swelling become. There are cases in which the ligament tears apart. This is a case for your doctor to diagnose.

This is the most common of all the injuries that can cause inflammation. These usually happen when your ankle buckles, causing all of your body weight to fall on your ankle. You can also sprain a knee. All sprains you can elevate the body part; ice down the area, and use a compress.

Sprained ankle

This is usually caused when you have landed wrong on your foot, making twist and leading to all your body weight landing on your ankle. You need to elevate the ankle to reduce the amount of blood flowing to the area.

Cold wrap:

- 12 drops of Basil Essential oil
- 36 Drops of Lavender Essential oil
- ¼ tablespoons Grapeseed oil
- ¾ c Sweet almond or Apricot Seed oil.
- 2 cups of warm water.

Mix the oils together and then whisk them into the water. Dampen a clean cloth with the water and wring until moist. Place it on the ankle under the ice pack. Leave on for half an hour.

If you have realized that heat makes the muscles relax, use 10 drops of cinnamon essential oil and 26 drops of Lavender. Place the cloth on the ankle before placing the heating pad. Replace the cloth after twenty minutes.

When you use the essential oils in this manner, you are keeping them in the affected area. This speeds the healing process. Using warm water activates the essential oils so they are working as soon as you apply the compress to your skin.

SAFETY NOTE: if it is a severe sprain, substitute black pepper essential oils for the cinnamon. It is more effective in reducing severe inflammation.

Foot Soak:

- 6 drops of Lavender Essential oil
- 2 Drops of Peppermint Essential oil
- 2 Drops of Basil Essential oil
- 2 Drops of Black pepper essential oil
- 2 tablespoons Sweet Almond or Apricot Kernel oil
- ¼ Cup Sea Salts

Thoroughly mix all the oils before adding them to the sea salts. Add half of the sea salts to warm water and soak your ankle for twenty minutes.

If you are hypertensive, mix 1/8 cup each of borax and baking soda and add the essential oils to them before adding the mixture to water. Use only half of the mixture. This is enough for two treatments.

Elbows

A sprain of the elbow can come from overuse or over extension. Soaking elbows can be cumbersome and almost impossible. It is better to mix a lotion or poultice when you sprain a body part that cannot be soaked due to location. Massage oils can be used as liniment in these cases as well. Just remember to apply it as you would liniment. Do not massage the oils into the sprain. Massaging a sprained area can worsen the injury.

Massage oil:

- 2 tablespoons Sweet Almond or Apricot oil
- 4 Drops of Roman Chamomile Essential oil
- 2 Drops of Cinnamon bark essential oil
- 4 drops of Peppermint oil
- 2 drops of Lavender essential oil

Mix together well and apply to sprained area. Wrap area with a bandage to keep the oils from rubbing off. Reapply every four to six hours or until the swelling subsides.

Another thing you can do it adds this to a ¼ cup of water, soak the bandage in it and wring it out until it's damp. Wrap it around the elbow and place another bandage over the first to keep in the moisture.

Twisted/sprained knees

These happen during sporting events, overextending during exercise, and even doing projects around the home when you twist your leg slightly without turning your whole leg. Again, if the swelling is pronounced, meaning your knee is the size of a grapefruit or larger, go to the emergency room. This is a severe sprain or it may be the sign of a more serious knee injury. Again, elevate the leg and get an ice pack ready.

Sprained knee massage oil:

- 2 tablespoons of Sweet Almond or Apricot Kernel oil
- 3 drops of Sweet Marjoram
- 2 Drops Lavender
- 1 Drop Cinnamon

Mix all the ingredients together well, and rub lightly into the affected area. DON'T MASSAGE IT INTO THE SWOLLEN TISSUE. This can cause further injury. Rubbing lightly will still apply the oil where it is needed. On the skin it will be absorbed.

Sprained knee Compress:

- 4 tablespoons Sweet Almond or Apricot Kernel Oil
- 6 drops of Sweet Marjoram
- 4 Drops of French Basil
- 4 Drops of Black Pepper
- 6 Drops of Lavender
- 4 Drops of Peppermint
- ½ cup of warm water

Mix all the oils together, and then add to the warm water. Place the cloth in the water. Wring it out until it is damp, and then apply it to the knee before the ice pack. Stay off of the knee as much as possible. This may mean using crutches until you can put weight on it. Until then, bend and straighten the knee a total of 30 times each day to keep optimum function of the knee. This is broken down into three sets of ten with a five-second break between each set.

All sprains need to be lightly exercised. This just means moving the area around to keep it loosened up. This will prevent stiffness and atrophy from lack of use during the recovery process.

Chapter 5: Carpal Tunnel

Ever since people have used their hands to knit, crochet, write for extended periods of time and even type, this ailment has reared its ugly head. The nerve cluster in your wrist shoots pain into your fingers along with tingling and swelling, which makes any kind of activity involving manual dexterity impossibility. People that twist their wrists repeatedly, as in making wire art, have a chance in getting this as well.

It happens when the same ligaments and tendons to the same action over and over, causing them to be strained and this causes swelling. This can happen to elbows as well (Tennis Elbow).

Avoid bending the wrists when the pain is present. You can lightly apply pressure to the base of the wrist in small circles. This soothes the nerves in the wrist and can alleviate some pain.

For injuries of this nature, add these essentials oil to your list:

Lemongrass (Cymbopogon citratus)

- This essential oil has proven to be a miracle worker.
- It helps to rebuild ligaments, tendons, and other connective tissues.

PATCH TEST IS HIGHLY RECOMMENDED WITH LEMONGRASS. IT CAN IRRITATE THE SKIN.

Palmarosa (Cymbopogon martini)

-   This essential oil helps to speed up recovery time by promoting cell regeneration.

Carpal Tunnel Oil:

-   1 tablespoon of Sweet Almond or Apricot seed oil
-   1 teaspoon of Grapeseed Oil
-   3 Drops of Black Pepper
-   2 Drops of lavender
-   2 Drops of Lemongrass
-   2 Drops of Palmarosa

Mix all of these together and massage into the centre of the wrist half an inch below the palm of the hand. This is where the major nerve cluster is for the hand. Massaging this mixture into the wrist will help to restore the tissues, alleviate pain, and help to get rid of the tingling in the fingers and even the numbness.
When you sleep at night, it is highly recommended that you wear wrist splints or braces that do not allow the wrists to bend during sleep. Before you place these on your wrists, apply the oil.

Warm Wrap:

-   2 tablespoons of a pepper infused oil, preferably cayenne
-   4 drops of Lemongrass
-   4 drops of Palmarosa
-   4 drops of peppermint

- ¼ cup of warm salt water (With sea salt)

Mix all the ingredients together and soak a sports bandage in it. Wring it out until it is moist and wrap the wrist with it. You can cover this with another wrap to keep the moisture from leaving. You can place a heating pad on it as well. If not using the heating pad, replace when is cold. If using a heating pad, replace every two hours.

Both recipes can be used on the elbow injury as well. The elbow must be kept in a bent position to minimize pain. Check range of motion for the elbow periodically and visit the emergency room if the injury worsens.

Chapter 6: Breathing Better

No one ever thinks about it. Your nose is stuffy so you blow it. The problem is when you blow your nose, nothing comes onto the tissue, but you still can't breathe. This is due to inflammation. Your sinusitis has inflamed the tissues in your sinus cavities causing your nasal passages to be constricted. If this is you, add these to the basic list in chapter 3:

Eucalyptus (Eucalyptus globulus)

- Clears blocked passages and helps to rid the respiratory system of infections.
- Has been used to treat sinusitis, asthma, and bronchitis, as well as throat infections.
- It can soothe coughs as well.

Clove (Syzygium aromaticum)

- It has antibacterial properties to help eliminate infection.
- Helps asthmatics and bronchitis sufferers breathe better by opening airways.
- If you have sensitive skin, this essential oil is not recommended for your use. It can cause skin irritation and dermatitis.

Lemon (Citrus lemon)

- It has strong antibacterial properties which can eliminate infections.
- Can bring down fevers in cases of sinus infections
- Helps to relieve tightness in the chest and inflammation due to sinus and lung infections.
- A patch test is recommended for this one as it can cause skin irritation.

Rosemary (Rosmarinus officinalis)

- Can help treat asthma and bronchitis attacks.
- Can soothe inflamed alveoli and sinus cavities.
- Is recommended for use in place of Eucalyptus for children. It's milder.
- Do not use if you are pregnant, hypertensive, or suffer from epilepsy.

DON'T APPLY ANY MASSAGE OILS DIRECTLY TO THE EYES. THE ESSENTIAL OILS CAN CAUSE EYE IRRITATION.

Respiratory mineral bath:

- ¼ cup Borax
- ¼ cup baking soda
- ½ cup fine Sea Salt or Ground Steel Cut oats if you are hypertensive.
- ¼ cup Sweet Almond or Apricot Seed oil
- 6 drops Rosemary

- 4 drops Lavender
- 4 drops Peppermint
- 4 drops Cinnamon
- 4 Drops Eucalyptus (If administering to a child, increase the peppermint by this amount)
- 2 Drops Clove

Mix all the dry ingredients first. Mix all the oils separate from the dry ingredients. Mix the dry ingredients into the oils and let sit in a tightly lidded container overnight. Add half of the mixture to warm running water and bath as normal.

Use a quarter of the amount for children 4 to 10 years of age.

Because of the Lavender and Rosemary, this can be done before bed.

Diffuser Mix:

- 4 Drops of Rosemary
- 4 Drops of Lavender
- 2 drops of lemon

Mix together and place 5 drops on a plug-in diffuse pad or potpourri bowl. As it gently heats, it will release the scents making breathing easier and aiding in sleep.

Chest Rub:

- ½ cup of Sweet Almond oil or Apricot Seed oil
- 10 drops of Sweet Basil

- 10 drops of Rosemary or Eucalyptus
- 10 drops of Lavender
- 5 drops of lemon
- 5 drops of peppermint
- 2 drops of clove
- 7 drops of Black pepper

Mix all ingredients together and rub into the chest area. This can be done before bed even though there are stimulants in it. This will help open up the chest, reduce lung inflammation and facilitate sleep.

For Sinuses: Rub into the brow line, along the bridge of the nose to the cheek bones. This must be done in downward strokes and keeping the oils away from the eyes and eyelids.

Room Spray:

This can be used to kill the infection on surfaces and in the air. The mixture will also help breathing.

- ½ cup warm water
- 15 drops of Eucalyptus or peppermint
- 10 drops of Lavender
- 5 drops of Clove

Mix together in a spray bottle or mister. Shake well before spraying into the air.

While the illness is onset, do not over exert yourself, especially in the case of asthma or bronchitis. Strenuous aerobic exercises can lead to attacks where you are short of breath and even wheezing. Also avoid whole wheat products and milk products. They produce mucous in the system that can lead to flare-ups with bronchitis and sinusitis. Any strong seasoning combinations such as anything blackened can also provoke an attack.

This doesn't mean you can't exercise.

Start slow, listening to your body and learning its cues. Consult with your healthcare provider for approved exercises that you can when you start to exercise. In many cases of asthma and bronchitis, lung strength and capacity can be increased when taught proper breathing techniques.

Exercises that focus on breathing are highly recommended. Two of these exercises are Yoga and Tai Chi. You can also ask your doctor about Qi Gong. That is also a moving meditation that can strengthen your lungs.

Alternate nostril breathing can help relieve sinus issues. Neti pots come highly recommended as well, but when starting out with these, seek help from a professional that can properly train you in its use.

Chapter 7: Arthritis

That stiffness in the joint area and swelling of the joints can be due to the onset of arthritis. This can be through a trauma to the joints repeatedly over time or due to heredity. There are two types of arthritis. Osteoarthritis, the most common of the two, brings with it stiff and painful joints, and swelling as well. You feel stiff in the morning and it loosens up with a little activity only to get worse as the day goes on. Rain tends to aggravate it, and so does any changes in the outside pressure.

Keeping moving is the key to keeping the joints loose, but it's a battle when you are already in pain from joints that don't want to cooperate. You're tired because of the pain, and even though anti-inflammatory drugs help, they often need a little boost because they tend to wane before your next dose. This is due to cartilage damage from it wear thin between the joints. Rheumatoid arthritis is the second type and more severe of the two. It can often be completely debilitating, and often requires the sufferer to be in a wheel chair or rocker.

The body is openly attacking the body's tissues, and the person is often fatigued, in pain, and has very pronounced swollen joints.

Heat generally helps the joints loosen up enough to be able to move them, and avoiding foods in the nightshade family will help to prevent some swelling and discomfort:

- Potatoes
- Tomatoes

- Peppers
- Goji berries
- Eggplant.

All these vegetables and fruits contain enzymes that can bring on an attack or instigate one if swelling and pain isn't present. Other foods have been discovered to do the same, but it has been on a case by case basis. Find the foods that trigger attacks and eliminate them from your diet.

Kobumcha tea has also been known to help treat rheumatoid arthritis. The vitamins, minerals and enzymes present make the perfect combination for the treatment of arthritis as a whole.

Treating both forms of arthritis with essential oils is normally done with making salves and liniments, but to keep it simple; I will provide recipes that don't require extra ingredients or equipment. To specifically treat osteoarthritis, you need to narrow down your essential oils list to the following:

Juniper (Juniperus communis)

- This essential oil comes highly recommended for all types of arthritis.
- It removes toxins from the blood to help with the pain associated with the disorder, and also reduces swelling of the joints.
- Do not use if you are pregnant or suffering from kidney diseases.

Ginger (Zingiber officinalis)

- This essential oil specifically targets the fatigue that comes from dealing with the chronic pain of arthritis.
- It also reduces the aches and pains associated with the swelling.
- In a blend, it boosts the actions of other essential oils, making the blend more potent.

Frankincense (Boswellia carteri)

- This oil is highly touted for its ability to reduce inflammation.
- It also acts as a mild analgesic, reducing pain.

EVEN THOUGH THESE ARE LISTED FOR ARTHRITIS, THEY CAN ALSO BY USE IN ANY CASE OF INFLAMMATION, CHRONIC JOINT OR MUSCLE PAIN.

Body Butter for joints:

(I am using this instead of an ointment because body butter takes longer to absorb into the skin which lengthens the time the oils are in contact with the area.)
There are 4 ounces of fragrance Avocado or Shea Body Butter. You can mix the two if you like.

- 10 Drops of Frankincense
- 10 Drops of Juniper
- 10 Drops of Eucalyptus
- 5 Drops of Black Pepper
- 5 drops of Cinnamon
- 5 Drops of Lavender
- 5 Drops of Sweet Basil

Place all the ingredients in a mixing bowl and blend it on low speed for 3 minutes making sure none of the body butter is along the sides. Place the mixture in a container with a tight lid.

To use, rubs into the affected area as needed. If using before bed, wrap a bandage around joints such as knees and elbows. Cover hand with white gloves. Wrapping the affected parts ensures that the oils will not rub off during sleep. This makes the treatment more effective.

Full Body Soak:

- ½ cup coarse Sea Salt or ground Steel Cut Oats
- 1/8 cup Borax
- 1/8 cup Baking soda
- 1/8 Cup Grapeseed oil
- 1/8 Cup Sweet Almond or Apricot Kernel Oil
- 10 drops of Lavender
- 5 Drops of Juniper
- 5 Drops of Ginger
- 5 Drops of Frankincense

Mix the dry ingredients first, making sure they are completely mixed. Now, mix the oils. Mix the dry ingredients into the oils and make sure it is mixed well. Store tightly lidded container overnight. Use half of the mixture by pouring into a warm to slightly hot bath. This makes two treatments.

Joint Massage oil:

When the massaging aching joints, and do not dig into the affected areas with your hands. This will make the pain worse. Start by lightly rubbing the oil into the skin and gently apply pressure every ten minutes of the massage.

- 3 ounces of Sweet Almond or Apricot Kernel oil
- 1 ounce of Grapeseed Oil
- 10 Drops of Juniper oil
- 10 Drops of Ginger Oil
- 10 Drops of Peppermint Oil
- 5 Black Pepper Oil
- 5 Drops of Lavender Oil
- 5 Drops of Frankincense Oil
- 5 Drops of Clove oil

Mix all oils together and place it in a dark glass container with a tight lid. Store it in a dark cool place. Rub into the affected joints as needed to treat inflammation and general pain. If you use this before bed, wrap the treated area with a bandage, or, if applying to your hands, cover them with white cotton gloves.

Supplements

There are also many supplements, vitamin, mineral, and herbal that you can take as well to help swell of the joints and to speed healing:

Vitamins C and E

- These two works in conjunction with one another to help your body mend and regenerate connective tissue.
- They can help you bounce back from injuries quicker.
- While healing from an injury take 10k mcg of Vitamin C and 1000 mcg of vitamin E. This will give you the boost your body needs to recover.

Glucosamine and Chondroitin

- These two together have been proven to improve joint movement by reducing swelling and helping the body's natural healing process to restore full joint ability.
- Talk to your doctor about the dosage.

Devil's Claw

- Though the name is ominous, this herb comes highly recommended in holistic circles for all who suffer from arthritis.
- It reduces swelling, relieves pain, and also helps the body rebuild eroded tissue.

Ashwaganda Root

- This herb focuses on bringing your body into balance which helps it stops attacking it in autoimmune disease cases. It finds the root cause of the attack and corrects it. Mixed it the herb mentioned above, it is a veritable one-two punch for the treatment and managing of arthritis symptoms.

Carpal Tunnel-Avoiding surgery

Most cases of carpal tunnel end in costly and painful surgeries to the wrists. Surgery can be avoided if you use the blends above, and even learn to make your own. Take periodic breaks during the day to let your wrists rest.

Don't forget to wear your braces during rest periods. You can even place the oil blends on wrist wraps while you work to treat carpal tunnel as you work. If your fingers start tingle, stop work immediately. Don't work through the pain. This will only make it worse. Take the time needed to massage the nerves, treat the affected wrist(s), and then, when the tingling stops, continue working. Trying to work through the pain isn't showing a valiant effort, and can make carpal tunnel severe enough to warrant surgery.

Sprains

Most advice will have you walking on sprained ankles and trying to work as usual. This can worsen a sprain. Instead, gradually get it used to your weight and keep moving it sprained area periodically.

Our bodies are made to move, and when an area can't move for long periods of time, it becomes stiff and, in many cases, freeze, not being able to be used. I know it hurts to move it, but small motions will help keep the sprained area loosened up enough to be mobile when it heals.

Track your symptoms

In the cases of chronic inflammation, track your symptoms on a day-to-day basis. This means keeping a diary of what you have eaten and your body's reaction to it. If you are experiencing pain that is worse than normal, write it down. If you are having a great day, you need to track that as well. Also write down what you took it terms of medications and supplements. Enter in your diary any aromatherapy treatments as well.

Be candid with your doctor

Let them know your concerns. It's your body. Ask as many questions as you can when he or she is explaining treatments or new medications. Take your diary with you and let them look at it. This will help them immensely when they are adjusting prescriptions, adding new ones or deciding that you need to be taking off some of them. Don't be afraid to let them know if you are uncomfortable with a treatment they are prescribing.

If you have immediate reactions to anything, natural or prescribed, stop taking the treatment or supplement and make an appointment with your specialist as soon as possible. Don't wait and keep taking it. It could cause further complications and even make you develop another illness. All of these oils can be used in any case of inflammation. They all will work together to bring down inflammation while reducing the pain and stiffness of the injury. Clove and cinnamon oils should be used in small quantities as they are very potent and can cause harm in large doses.

If you are allergic to any of the plants forms of the oils listed above, leave the oil out of the recipe and substitute another on the list. The goal is to manage your pain and reduce swelling, and you can do this effectively without causing further discomfort. I hope the information in this book serves you well, and will help you become pain-free.

Last Words

Of all the essential oils listed above, the only one that is safe to use without diluting is Lavender. In a pinch, you can place a few drops on an inflamed area to soothe the ache of the joint and to start bringing down the swelling until you can make the blends above. Only use it sparingly. Your body can develop sensitivity to any essential oil if it is used repeatedly.

www.ingramcontent.com/pod-product-compliance
Lightning Source LLC
Chambersburg PA
CBHW072018280526
45788CB00007B/2593